Early Passage

A Journal for Parents of Premies

Priscilla Hernandez Hacker, PhD
and
Carolyn Ringo, RN, MSW

NICU INK®
BOOK PUBLISHERS
SANTA ROSA, CALIFORNIA

Editor-in-Chief:
Charles Rait, RN, MSEd, PNC

Managing Editor:
Suzanne G. Rait, RN

Editorial Coordinator:
Tabitha Parker

Editors:
Patricia Heinicke, Jr
Sylvia Stein Wright, BA

Proofreader:
Joanne Gosnell, BA

Book Design and Composition by
Marsha Godfrey Graphics

Edward Robert Hughes
Night with Her Train of Stars
Birmingham Museums & Art Gallery
Birmingham, England

NICU INK®
BOOK PUBLISHERS
1410 Neotomas Avenue, Suite 107
Santa Rosa, CA 95405-7533

LIBRARY OF CONGRESS CATALOGING-IN-PUBLICATION DATA
Hacker, Priscilla Hernandez, 1958–
Early passage : a journal for parents of premies / Priscilla Hernandez Hacker and Carolyn Ringo.
p. cm.
Includes bibliographical references.
ISBN 1-887571-08-6
1. Parents—Psychology—Miscellanea. 2. Parent and infant—Miscellanea. 3. Infants (Premature)—Miscellanea. 4. Diaries—Authorship. I. Ringo, Carolyn, 1955– II. Title.
HQ755.8 .H33 2001
306.874—dc21 2001032951

ISBN 1-887571-08-6

Table of Contents

For He will give His angels charge concerning you,
to guard you in all your ways.
They will bear you up in their hands,
lest you strike your foot against a stone.

(Psalms 91:11–12)

Acknowledgments

We are indebted to the following persons who have contributed to the making of this book in their own unique and invaluable way:

Thank you to our parent-reviewers who graciously shared of their time, their experiences, and their insight: Michol Ann Jensen (mom to Tilitha, 28 weeker, now eight years old) our home town editor; Sally Poutiatine (mom to Hailey, 28 weeker, now 18 months); Sara Groenheide (mom to Becky, 28 weeker, now three years old); Charlene Rathbun (mom to Cecily, 28 weeker, now two years old); Shannon Richards (mom to Andrew and Caleb, 28 weekers, now six years old); Teresa Dodge (mom to Emily Rose, 28.5 weeker, now two and a half); Michelle Dennison (mom to Lee, 28 weeker, now three and a half); Tracy Persing (mom to Stephen, 33 weeker, now four and a half, with multiple medical problems and global delays); Inge Gray (mom to 34.5 weeker twins, James now two and a half, and angel Spencer); Lisa Hairston (mom to Emily, now three years old); Alison Batchelder (mom to Joshua, six years old with significant complications); and Ed and Laurel Martinelli (parents to Buddy, 24 weeker, 2/22/97–7/12/97).

Thank you to Dr. Michael Barsotti, MD, for his expertise and encouragement.

Thank you to Mara Tesler Stein, PsyD (mom to Gavrielle and Layla, 30.5 weekers, now four and a half), for encouraging our work, and to the members of Preemie-L, an online support group for parents of premies, for sharing their own premie journeys.

Thank you to Y. Phoebe Hafersat, Debi Rowberg, and David Holt, PhD, who in reviewing the manuscript guided us with wisdom and encouragement. Thanks to Samuel I. Hernandez for technical support at all hours.

Many thanks to Phoebe Villalpanda and Leroy and Lura Hacker for support on the home front with cooking, cleaning, and caring for kids.

And last but not least, special thanks to Chuck Rait, who needed no convincing that this work was needed.

Introduction

As a clinical psychologist, I am familiar with the pain, sorrow, and confusion common to the human race. My own life challenges and those of my clients have taught me much about the human spirit's ability to cope and its courage to carry on.

However, nothing I had faced in my life prepared me for the roller coaster I was about to board when the birth of my son came three and a half months early. Despite my clinical training and years of walking alongside my clients with their struggles, I found myself overwhelmed with a flood of emotions, unable to sort them out on my own.

This specially formatted journal is designed to help parents like myself cope with the emotional turmoil of the various stages of the premie journey. Chapter by chapter, you will be able to explore your emotions, reactions, and experiences, with fill-in-the-blank sections provided to serve as prompts.

You may find specific sections of this journal especially helpful; others may not be relevant or pertinent to your particular journey. For instance, although some sections by their very nature will be specific to mothers, this journal is written for fathers as well. Feel free to complete those chapters or sections that address your particular needs while leaving other sections blank. Additionally, you may find that because your experience with premie-related issues changes over time, you may need to revisit and rework that with which you had previously made peace. You may find it helpful to return to the various chapters of this journal throughout the passage of your premie journey. Although the term *baby* is used for brevity's sake, consider it as referring to *babies* if you were blessed with multiple births.

As you work through this journal, you may find yourself experiencing painful emotions. Our intent is to assist you in facing, moving through, and coming to peace with your emotions. It is our hope and prayer that your journey through this book will bring healing. If in the course of completing this journal you find yourself needing additional assistance in coping with various premie-related issues, please refer to the resource section found in Appendix D or seek out a qualified mental health professional.

Health providers and others working with parents of premies may find this journal a useful tool in helping to direct parents through the emotional turmoil that comes with delivering and caring for these children. As parents work through the difficult and distressing feelings that come with having a premature baby, issues of loss, grief, anger, and resolution can develop into adaptation and strength.

Priscilla Hernandez Hacker

Dedication

To Matthew Daniel (my gift from God), whose early birth and resilience spurred the creation of this book, to Zachary David (God's blessing), who makes my heart sing, and to John (my strong arm), for the fullness of life you all bring to me.

Priscilla Hernandez Hacker

To all the parents whose love, patience, suffering, and endurance remind me what a precious gift life is and how grateful I am for my own two children, Liv and Nils.

Carolyn S. Ringo

Chapter 1
In The Beginning: We're Pregnant

Few preterm babies give notice in the first trimester that things will go awry in the months ahead. In these early months, mothers may be concerned about miscarriage, but they are usually not worrying about early delivery. And once they are past this initial phase, they often sigh in relief. In the second trimester, joyful anticipation of completing the pregnancy replaces earlier anxieties. This is often described as the time when pregnant women "radiate" and "bloom." They are usually beyond morning sickness and fatigue and may be pleased they are now starting to show. They have begun purchasing maternity clothes, and they may have a renewed interest in sexual activity. Overall, they have begun to feel good again.

Parents inclined to record the beginning of their baby's life don't have to look far to find a vast array of pregnancy calendars and journals. This is a precious time, worth remembering, and it makes sense that we want to record every detail.

However, when the normal course of pregnancy is interrupted and parents are ushered into the early passage of their premie journey, many things come to a screeching halt. The pregnancy calendar or journal, already filled with earlier entries, may be left incomplete. But the story doesn't end there, and it deserves completion in its own right, just as every full-term pregnancy does.

You may want to go back to that pregnancy calendar or journal to complete your or your partner's pregnancy story, or you may choose to use this chapter to recall and record the first phase of this pregnancy.

How did this pregnancy come to be? Was it a surprise or planned? Did you battle with infertility? If so, how was this resolved?

When I first suspected I was pregnant, I…

The way I found out I was pregnant was…

I let my partner know I was pregnant by…

I shared the news of my pregnancy with others by…

They responded by…

Becoming pregnant (or my partner's pregnancy) made me feel…

Were you ever concerned about miscarriage?

Did you have regular prenatal checkups and screenings? If yes, describe these.

Did you alter your diet or lifestyle in any way? If so, how?

Were you considered high-risk? If so, why?

Did you have ultrasounds or amniocentesis? What was this experience like for you and your partner?

Did you know the sex of your baby? What plans did you begin to make, if any, as a result of this information?

Describe how you felt physically and emotionally during your first trimester.

Looking back, what I remember most about my first trimester was…

How did your thoughts and feelings change as you entered each new trimester?

Notes

Chapter Two
Interrupted Pregnancy

A support group for mothers with premies in the NICU gathered to share their experiences and concerns. Although their babies had been born prematurely for a variety of reasons, one common experience these moms described was the difficulty in letting go of their pregnancy. Many spoke of their pain and even tears in seeing pregnant women. Their empty wombs, in contrast to the "full and bulging" look of women still pregnant, represented a loss. The ideal pregnancy, the one that would culminate in a planned labor and delivery, yielding a bouncy baby, had slipped out of their reach. This was not to be their story. Moms who had been hospitalized for weeks of bed rest spoke of their desire to "just have this baby now," and of their guilt for having had those thoughts. These moms, along with those who had no forewarning, were all grieving the loss of a pregnancy they had so much wanted to continue. Statements such as "I just wasn't ready to not be pregnant" and "I wanted to still have my baby inside of me" expressed common sentiments.

In addition to the loss of their pregnancies, many moms shared the painfully common experience of wondering what they had done to cause their baby's early delivery. Searching for answers often led to a variety of further questions. "Was it the thoughts I had about not wanting to deliver a big baby?" "Was it the exercise class I attended when I was tired?" "Was it the medication I took before I even knew I was pregnant?" An incompetent cervix, premature rupture of membranes, and infections are common causes of premature deliveries, but for many moms, the cause of their baby's premature birth will remain unknown. And it is the unknowns that often give moms the greatest amount of grief, perhaps because the unknown underscores the degree to which we have no control and our inability to ensure this will never happen again. As one mom shared, "My doctor said that probably the hardest thing for me would be that we just don't know what caused my preterm delivery, and we probably never would. I finally had to let go of my 'needing to know' because it just wasn't going to happen." Although there are always many questions, there are oftentimes too few answers.

In the mothers' group and beyond, we each have a need to tell our story. Describing our experience is especially helpful in dealing with those things we cannot make sense of and the things over which we have no control.

Perhaps you will find it helpful to write your own story.

I first suspected something was wrong when…

How were your suspicions confirmed, and what was your response? What was your partner's response?

Describe your third trimester (if the pregnancy lasted that long).

What happened when you or your partner first went into labor?

How did you react when you realized this was no dress rehearsal?

What questions or thoughts were spinning in your head, and with whom did you share these?

Did you get answers to your questions before your baby was born?

Describe the labor and delivery, including who attended your birth and your reaction to this experience.

What was your emotional reaction to your baby's premature delivery?

My partner responded to the baby's early arrival by…

Did you have time to take a childbirth education class or refresher course? How did this affect your experience of the baby's premature delivery?

Had you discussed a birthing plan with your partner and/or your doctor?

Who if anyone, did you blame when things didn't go as expected? Why?

When I first woke up after recuperating from my baby's birth, I...

When I first felt my abdomen and realized that my baby was not inside me, I...

If I stated or secretly wished my baby would come soon, I didn't mean…

If I said "I don't want a big baby," I didn't mean…

When was the first time you saw your baby? What was this like for you?

Not being able to see, hold, or feed my baby immediately after delivery made me feel…

Were you prepared for how small or underdeveloped your baby would be?

Did your baby have to be transported to another hospital?

Were you transported with your baby? What was this like for you emotionally?

During your hospitalization, did you experience discomfort with the maternity-ward noises of women in labor and the cries of newborns?

Was the hospital staff helpful to you during this time? If so, how?

Who was your main support, and how were they helpful?

Was anything said or done that was hurtful to you? What was it? What was your response?

What was the most critical element of your loss? How did you cope?

Did your mode of coping change over time? If so, how?

Many parents struggle with feeling both angry at their loss and guilty about having these feelings, because their baby is alive. Have you struggled with similar feelings?

If you were on long-term bed rest yet your pregnancy ended prematurely, did you experience a sense of failure, injustice, or helplessness? What other feelings did you experience? What was the most difficult aspect for you?

I had envisioned my baby's birth story to be…

About the actual birth, I felt…

Describe your reaction to being discharged without your baby

What did you feel when you were out in public without being pregnant and/or without your baby in tow?

When I first went home to the empty space that my baby would have filled, I felt…

If it was determined, what was the cause of your premature labor and delivery?

Did you feel that you were to blame for this condition?

What were your thoughts and emotional reactions to your diagnosis or the lack of one?

Although you probably weren't ready for your baby to come early, how did you start to get ready (mentally, physically, emotionally, spiritually) for the journey ahead?

Have you felt the desire, on some level, to have your baby back in your womb so you could finish your pregnancy?

What can you give your baby now that would represent what you were prevented from giving before by the earlier delivery?

Despite it all, were there ways in which you were grateful?

What would you say to help other premie parents—either something that was said to you or something you wished had been said?

Notes

Chapter Three
The Critical First 72 Hours

For most parents, the birth of their baby brings immense joy and gladness. For premie parents, their baby's early delivery comes with emotions at the opposite end of the spectrum. Sheer terror, disbelief, sadness, loss, and anger are among the early and sometimes enduring emotions premie parents experience. Resignation, then hope and courage follow quickly for some, but more slowly for others.

The range of precipitating factors contributing to the delivery of premature babies is vast. Yet most premie parents face concern about the immediate survival or long-term outcome for their baby. Their vision of how life would be after pregnancy becomes a fading mirage. In its place is the frightening reality of life in the NICU.

Depending upon their baby's condition, parents are often informed that the first 72 hours are the "most critical." There are no guarantees of survival for micropremies (those born 12 or more weeks premature) and only cautious predictions for babies who are older gestationally. Neonatologists report that during these early days, a baby's condition can change rapidly and acutely. Risk is at its highest during the first 72 hours. Many conditions, such as intraventricular hemorrhage (IVH), patent ductus arteriosus (PDA), and respiratory distress syndrome (RDS), to name a few, can develop.

During these first few days, it is too early for doctors to be able to know their premie patients and too soon for them to be able to predict how these fragile infants will respond. Generally speaking, it is not until after the first week of life that doctors are able to read the baby's responses and to conjecture about outcomes.

Thus, in this early period of a baby's life, the medical team can only speak of the here and now. Making projections, even into the near future, is unwise because it can set parents up for false expectations. All this ambiguity comes at a time when parents need, more than anything, some thread of hope to hang onto and some promise that all will be well. With their baby's life hanging in the balance, parents often feel that they are left hanging, too.

Consider your own experience during the early phase of your baby's NICU stay.

My reaction to my baby's NICU admittance was…

Did you know what to expect when you got to the NICU?

Were you prepared for your baby's size, condition, and appearance?
How did this affect you?

Were you prepared to see your baby attached to the IVs, wires, monitors, or other equipment?

My reaction to all the medical equipment was…

Describe your baby's first 72 hours of life.

What were your feelings and concerns during your baby's first few days in the NICU?

When I was told that the first 72 hours would be the most critical for my baby, I thought and felt…

What did you understand about this "critical" phase?

Were you ever concerned about your baby's survival? If so, did you share this with anyone?

I coped with the wait-and-see period of the first 72 hours by...

Did your baby survive?

Were you reassured at some point that your baby would live? How did this news change your emotional state?

Was your baby intubated (placed on a respirator)? If so, for how long? What were your reactions to this?

What were you told about RDS? Did you have any concerns about this condition?

Did your baby have IVH? If so, what level were these brain bleeds? What was your understanding of this condition? What was your reaction to your baby having this condition and to the risks associated with it?

Did your baby have PDA? Was he or she responsive to medication, or was surgery required?

Did your baby need blood transfusions? If so, how many? What was your reaction to this?

Were you informed about donating blood for your baby? Did a family member participate? Were there issues or concerns regarding blood transfusions or blood donations for your baby?

Did you have concerns about the invasiveness of the medical procedures necessary to keep your baby alive?

Who kept you informed of your baby's changing condition?

Were you satisfied with the explanations you received concerning your baby's condition?

With whom did you feel comfortable asking questions?

Did you get any emergency calls from the NICU doctors? Why did you get called? What was your reaction to these calls?

Were pain management issues ever addressed with you?

Were you ever informed of possible medication side effects? If so, did the information influence the medications your baby received?

Were questions of whether to stop medical treatments for your baby ever discussed? If so, what were your reactions to this discussion?

Were issues of the possible long-term consequences of prematurity addressed with you? What were you told? What was your reaction?

Notes

Notes

Notes

Chapter Four
Whose Baby Is This? Collaborative Care

When a baby is sent to the NICU, parents are filled with a sense of fear and trepidation. Understandably so, because only babies with critical health issues are granted admission. The NICU, with all its high-tech equipment, is also equipped with a high-tech staff. Neonatologists work on the cutting edge of their dynamic field. Nurses with state-of-the-art training work to care for these fragile babies around the clock. This setting can be comforting to parents who feel, and in actuality are, unable to care for the needs of their newborn. Although moms might wish their baby was still "cooking," "growing," and "thriving" within them and are grieved that this is not so, they report being thankful for the substitute womb-like environment of the NICU. Parents look to the nursing staff for instruction on how to facilitate bonding, how to "read" their infant's cues, and how to handle and care for their new and fragile bundle. For this training, they are indebted.

There comes a time, however, when this once comforting environment is transformed into an intrusive holding tank in the minds of many, if not most, premie parents. This change in mind-set often occurs when a premie has reached the feed-and-grow stage and has moved from being a "newbie" to being an "oldie-on-the-block." The shift can occur even before parents realize what has happened. And it is usually prompted by the actions of a hurried or oblivious nurse who is not yet aware that these parents are now ready to take on more care of their infant. This nurse might have changed a diaper, read a temperature, given a first bath, or completed a feeding while mom or dad waited outside the unit, ready and willing to provide this care. Perceiving that they have been usurped in their parental role can set parents into a stance of alarm and defensiveness, and resentment may follow because they have to "share" their baby with others over whom they have no control. It is at this point that moms will say to a supportive ear, "Whose baby is this, anyway?" One mom reported that close to the time of discharge, while holding her baby, she fought the impulse to run out the door and escape with him, thinking to herself, "Let's make a run for it!"

Moms and dads often say that it is difficult to feel like a "mom" or a "dad" when their baby is being cared for by others and must reside outside of their home. Having to wait until permission is granted to touch, hold, or diaper their infant goes against every grain of parenthood within. Yet, this is the reality of the NICU. Parents sometimes resent the very place responsible for saving their infant's life and the very people who administered life-saving care; this seeming contradiction creates its own unique stress. The NICU staff can be a strange set of bedfellows that parents can both resent and appreciate, be repelled by and drawn to, at the same time. It may be a relief for parents to recognize that this changing perception about the NICU is a normal part of the premie process. This understanding can help steady parents for the duration of their NICU stay, until the time when they are able to parent unencumbered.

As the date of discharge nears, a second transformation takes place for many premie parents. This time, a renewed appreciation for the nurses, doctors, and other medical staff who cared for their critically ill baby emerges. Although glad and relieved to be leaving the NICU, parents may also feel a sense of sadness and a new sense of loss at having to leave behind those people who collaboratively cared for their baby. It can be a comfort to parents to learn that the NICU staff also undergoes a similar transformation. As the need for collaborative care diminishes and the shift of care to parents nears, the staff experiences a sadness and sense of loss that they will soon be saying good-bye to the babies and parents they cared for.

Tell your story of collaborative care in the NICU.

Did you have difficulty feeling like your baby's mom or dad? If so, at what point did this change for you?

Was the medical staff instrumental in helping you nurture and parent your baby despite the limitations imposed by medical interventions? If so, how?

Did you find the nursing staff able to support whatever level of care you were able to give to your baby?

What was your response to needing to obtain "permission" to hold, feed, or care for your baby?

What was the staff's response to your role in your baby's care?

Was the staff sensitive to your changing needs as a parent in regard to your baby's care?

Was your baby's care ever in conflict with your desires (e.g., regarding breast- or bottle feedings, schedule of care, medications)?

Did you experience difficulty with the NICU visitation rules or schedules?

While already feeling the stress of having a premie, did you also experience conflict with anyone in particular on the NICU staff? If so, describe what happened.

How did you cope with this conflict? Were you able to voice your concerns or to insist that this individual be removed from your baby's care team? What was your emotional reaction?

Were there other issues about sharing your baby's care with the NICU staff with which you found yourself struggling? If so, how did you get help or support?

Did you find yourself becoming frustrated with the very place that was instrumental in your baby's survival?

Did you find yourself resenting the fact that your days in the NICU were not over yet?

What helped you steady your course until the race was run? How did you cope with the angst?

As the day of discharge drew near, did you find yourself doing an about-face? Did you fear that you weren't ready to take on full care of your baby and wish that you could take the nursing staff home with you?

Some parents, although they are glad to be leaving the NICU, also feel a sense of loss in leaving behind the nurses upon whom they have come to depend. Did you experience anything like this? If so, what helped you through this process?

Did you visit the NICU after your baby's discharge, or do you have plans to visit?

Knowing what you know now, what, if anything, do you wish had been different for you and your baby in the NICU?

Notes

Notes

Chapter Five
The NICU and the Waiting Game

A mother was describing her baby's delivery and immediate transfer to the NICU. Her daughter had been hospitalized for 11 days, yet in recounting her story, she said that her baby had been there for 11 months. When questioned about this, she replied, "For 11 months? Did I say months? Well, it sure seemed like that."

Whatever the length of your baby's stay in the NICU, it is always longer than you expected. Neonatal intensive care is not part of anyone's "birth plan."

Following their adjustment to the critical first few days of their premie's birth, parents begin to learn a new vocabulary and become immersed in a world for which they had little or no preparation. The first and most important question parents want to have answered is "When can I take my baby home?" But to this question there are rarely definite answers.

The NICU experience can feel like a waiting game, and parents soon settle in for the long haul. Even with all its machines, tubes, beeps, and smells, the NICU becomes a second home. Other sources of stress fade in comparison to the priority of their baby's health. The opportunities for hands-on care can become the most cherished moments of the day, and how parents feel is often a reflection of how their baby is doing. The waiting game continues. Parents experience the stress of waiting for the doctor's report each day and of bracing themselves each night for the doctor's dreaded call, which can only mean bad news. The core issue parents deal with is their need to know that their baby will survive.

Parents wait eagerly for the first time they can hold their baby, and some are resentful that they have to be given permission to do so. Mothers wait for the next time to pump their breasts, some hoping they will not be asked how much milk they got. Throughout this time, parents wait eagerly for their baby to be strong enough to take in a feeding of milk or formula, and then they hope their baby's digestive system is developed enough to tolerate the feeding. They wait for days free of apnea and bradycardia (As and Bs) and feel so helpless when their baby has another spell. Moms who work outside the home wait for direction about when to return to work, how much maternity leave to save for when the baby comes home, or whether to return to work at all. Those with children at home grapple with balancing visits to the NICU with their need to be home. Mostly, parents wait for word that the time to take their baby home has finally come. So much waiting, so many questions, and so few answers are the name of this game.

Ponder how the waiting game has been for you.

What were you told about how long your baby would need to stay in the NICU?

My reaction to this news was…

How long did you have to wait to:

See your baby?

Hold your baby?

Change your baby's diaper?

Feed your baby?

Bathe your baby?

Have your other children hold or feed their baby brother or sister?

How long did you have to wait for reassuring news about your baby?

How long did you have to wait to be certain of your baby's discharge date?

I coped with the long wait by…

What comforting words or actions were given to you during your baby's NICU stay?

How often were you at the hospital with your baby? Describe these visits and your response to them.

When I wasn't at the hospital, I thought and felt...

From whom did you receive support (physically, emotionally, financially, spiritually)?

In what ways did you feel most supported?

Were there things that others said or did that were hurtful to you?

How did you respond to the hurt?

In order to spend time at the hospital, what adjustments had to be made at home? How did these adjustments affect you and your family?

If you had prior medical or hospitalization experience, being thrust into the NICU may have triggered painful memories. How did you deal with these memories?

During your baby's stay in the NICU, were there other stressful circumstances in your life?

While my baby was in the NICU, I took care of myself and my partner by…

My partner took care of me by…

What were some of the high points during your baby's NICU stay?

Throughout the course of your baby's NICU stay, did your feelings change?

When the NICU staff first mentioned the word discharge, *my reaction was…*

How did you, or will you, celebrate the end of the waiting game?

Have you returned to visit the NICU since your baby's discharge? What emotions and memories were triggered from this visit?

If you haven't visited yet, do you plan to visit when your baby is strong enough to be out in public? How will you prepare yourself for the possibility of memories and emotions being triggered?

How do you hope this visit will go?

NOTES

Notes

Notes

Chapter Six

Facing Critical Illness and Surgery

Although the premie journey is often described as a roller coaster ride over which one has no control, perhaps the most turbulent time of all is when parents are informed that their premie is critically ill or in need of surgery. With advanced medical technologies, some parents know in advance, even before the birth, that their baby will need surgery. Others are caught totally by surprise. In either case, the news can be a crushing blow.

Nothing can prepare parents for the emotional tidal wave that overcomes them at the very time they need clear heads for making important decisions for their baby. The thought of one's tiny and fragile baby fighting a life-threatening illness or having to endure surgery is terrifying. Parents often ask "Why does she have to go through anymore?" "Hasn't he endured enough already?" "Will my baby survive the surgery?" "What if my baby dies?" If given the chance, most parents would gladly trade places with their baby. Their total dependence upon others to care for or even to save their baby can leave parents feeling completely helpless and at the mercy of the powers that be. Whether a baby's surgery is considered "major" or "minor," is planned or unplanned, it is a crisis that underscores just how little control parents have over the events that their baby must endure.

The hours during surgery or other critical periods can be emotionally draining, as moms and dads await words of reassurance or signs of healing. This process is equally intense for parents who live far from the hospital. These parents must communicate with doctors via telephone to discuss options for their baby and to provide consent. Whatever the case, parents face wrenching emotions that may churn within for a long time.

At times like these, moms and dads need to summon all the resources available to them. Family, friends, and faith can be essential emotional and spiritual supports, and these are desperately needed.

Sometimes parents are grateful that their baby was not born 20 years earlier, and they find hope in state-of-the-art medical technology. Or they trust in God and take courage as their faith and hopes are challenged and strengthened.

Recount your experience of your baby's critical illness or surgery.

How did you first come to know of your baby's critical illness and/or need for surgery?

What kind of preparation did you have for this news? What were your thoughts and feelings?

I coped with my baby's critical illness and/or need for surgery by…

While my baby was in surgery, I coped with the wait by…

Who was with you during your baby's most critical hours or days, and how did they show support?

What was your greatest fear at the time? Did you share this fear with anyone?

When I first saw my baby after surgery, I felt…

To me, my baby appeared…

Standing beside the isolette, I wanted to tell my baby…

What were signs of hope to you?

Did you blame anyone or anything for your baby's condition?

If your baby needed to be transferred to another facility for surgery or care, what was your response to this?

What preparations or arrangements did you need to make to be with your baby?

If you have older children, what and how did you tell them about their sibling's condition? How did they respond?

If you were not able to be present during your baby's surgery, how did you feel about this?

Some babies need multiple surgeries or have continued setbacks. If this was true for your baby, how did you deal with the ups and downs?

How did you gather information about your baby's condition? Was it through doctors, other hospital staff, friends, other premie parents, books, or Internet sites? Who or what was most helpful?

Often parents learn from their children. What has your baby taught you through all of this?

Notes

Notes

Chapter Seven

Hopes Deferred: Grieving the Death of Your Baby

When parents have a premature baby, thoughts and fears of losing their baby are inescapable. Although most premie parents will never experience the worst of these fears, for those who do, their world is changed forever. Suddenly they are robbed of their new baby's life and of so many hopes and dreams. In its wake are disappointments—some that are known and can be verbalized and others that are buried deep within. Death deals a heavy blow to the normal expectation that children will outlive their parents. When a premature baby dies, whether quickly, unexpectedly, after a prolonged battle for life, or in spite of numerous medical interventions, the reality and impact of the loss are devastating.

For some parents, the pain is compounded when they are asked to make a decision to withdraw life support for their baby. This is one of the hardest decisions anyone could be asked to make. Although choosing to withdraw life support may be the most loving and compassionate thing parents can do, it can still feel like a crushing blow. Yet, however heartrending death is, seeing and holding their baby during or just after death can be very healing for parents and can help them accept the painful reality of their loss. One mom said, "I will be forever grateful that I could be with her in her last moments and that I was able to hold her and tell her how much I loved her. It greatly comforted me to know that she wasn't afraid when she passed on." In addition to saying good-bye, having pictures and keepsakes of your baby can also bring about healing. They become priceless reminders to parents, siblings, and others that their baby remains a part of their lives.

As parents begin to adapt to the loss of their baby, they may experience a broad range of emotions in their grieving process. At times, life seems out of balance and somewhat surreal as simple decisions become overwhelming, focusing becomes more difficult, and routine enjoyments no longer bring happiness. Moms find that even their body does not cooperate, as it continues to produce milk, unable to recognize that the baby has died. Some parents may feel angry and betrayed by the universe, blaming God or others, or they may simply ask in resignation "Why me?" Few parents escape without some lingering feelings of guilt. Though the physiological and emotional responses may vary, it is important to note that over time symptoms of depression may follow the death of one's baby.

Parents often anticipate and feel a sense of pain and dread as the anniversary dates of their baby's birth and death draw near. It is common for friends and family to forget these occasions, but they remain significant to parents. Anticipating these times and planning ways to nurture yourself, your spouse, and your other children will help ease the pain. Planning something special to remember your baby can bring meaning to an otherwise mournful event. Some parents contribute flowers at their place of worship to commemorate their baby's death. Others make contributions to charity.

The first holidays after the baby's death may also be intensely difficult. One dad described his family's first Christmas following the death of their baby as "awful," recalling that they grappled with questions such as "Do we put out another stocking or not?" Family pictures that include the deceased child understandably reinforce the feeling that someone is missing. This sense of loss is likely most poignant during the holidays. Advance discussion about what traditions to keep and what new ones to begin may be a welcome solution. One family decided to "light a special candle in memory of [their] baby and make an ornament each year to hang on [their] tree to remember him."

There is no magical time frame for healing a broken heart. Pain and loss lead parents to hope for a magic formula that will quickly alleviate their grief and agony. However, grief is a long process. Even when parents begin to feel "normal" again, a familiar song, scent, or setting can ambush them, triggering sad memories and dormant grief. There is no quick fix for grief, but time, self-expression, sharing with others, and physical exercise will all help to restore wholeness again. In the end, perseverance through the grief process restores hope in the future and renews joy. With the passage of time, parents eventually come to accept their loss. One dad shared, "I will tell you, it gets easier over time. One day you will be happy again. One day you will find joy in things, and one day you will laugh again and not betray the memory of your child by being happy. It's been almost 1,000 days since Buddy left, and I've thought of him at least once every day, sometimes with joy and sometimes in pain."

Record the journey of your own grief process.

How were you told of your child's imminent death? Were you prepared for the news? If so, how were you prepared?

Did you request a second opinion about your baby's condition? Was this helpful? If so, in what way?

How did you deal with the reality that your baby would die?

What was your partner's response to this reality?

In what ways did you prepare for your baby's death? Who was there to help you?

Describe the end of your baby's life.

Were you able to say good-bye to your baby? If so, how did you do this? If not, is there anything you'd like to say or do now to say good-bye?

Was your partner involved in saying good-bye?

What did you do or say that was especially important to you in those final moments?

Were you able to hold your baby when he or she died? What are your memories of these moments?

Who was with you when your baby died?

How did your other children learn about the death of their sibling? How did they respond?

Who was available to provide comfort to your children?

Were your other children involved in saying good-bye?

Losing a child can put a strain on parents' relationships as each one is overwhelmed with his or her own grief. Parents can find themselves unable to lean on their partner or to meet each other's needs. Does this describe your situation? If so, how?

Sometimes partners can be angry at the other's reactions or feel the need to be strong for or take care of the partner. Did you feel this way? If so, how was this demonstrated?

Throughout the ordeal of my baby's illness and death, my main source of strength was…

At the time of my baby's death, what I needed most was…

I was able to get my needs met by…

Do you have a faith or religious affiliation? Has this had any bearing on how you coped with your baby's death?

Does your belief system offer you hope or comfort?

Feelings of jealousy and anger are normal. Seeing others with healthy thriving babies or viewing advertisements for baby products can trigger these emotions. Have you had this experience?

Sometimes parents become overprotective of their surviving children after the death of their baby. Have you had this experience? If so, describe what you were feeling and what happened as a result.

Often even simple tasks, such as cleaning house, shopping for groceries, and attending public functions, can seem overwhelming. Have you struggled with these tasks?

How have you coped with daily tasks that may now seem meaningless in comparison to dealing with death?

In the early days following my baby's death, the most helpful thing was…

Even more helpful would have been…

Sometimes people say unhelpful things or make poor comparisons to loss in their own life. Has this happened to you? If so, describe what was said and how you reacted.

What would have been more helpful? How would you like people to respond when you mention your baby's death?

Even though it is difficult to understand or admit, many parents feel some anger toward their baby for leaving them. Others feel guilt or even a sense of relief. Many experience various combinations of all of these feelings. Is anger toward your baby an emotion you have felt? If so, what is this anger about?

Recognizing feelings of guilt can be an important step toward healing. Do you feel any guilt about your baby's illness and/or death?

Do you feel a sense of relief for your baby or for yourselves? If so, describe this feeling.

Do you feel a need to express forgiveness to your baby?

Do you feel a need to ask forgiveness of your baby?

Do you feel a need to receive forgiveness from others, such as your partner?

The baby's due date, birthday, and death date, along with family holidays, can stir memories and emotions. Have you had this experience?

During these times, I have cared for myself, my spouse, and my other children by…

I have commemorated (or will commemorate) my baby's anniversary dates by…

The lingering questions I still ask myself about my baby's death are…

Does your baby's death cause you concern about having more children?

Notes

Notes

Chapter Eight
Spiritually Speaking

William Thomas Cummings once said, "There are no atheists in the fox holes."* For parents facing the untimely birth of their baby, the sense of helplessness that often accompanies this crisis can leave them feeling as though they have been dropped into a big pit. Standing by, powerless, as their baby wages the battle for life compels parents to search their souls and to grasp onto that which promises help and strength. Some parents find hope in "signs" that they believe mean something about their baby's outcome. They report finding peace in the meaning ascribed to a rainbow, a raven, a vision of an angel, or an encouraging scripture verse.

Parents who enter the premie journey with a strong sense of God's presence in their lives report finding peace in the knowledge that their plight is part of God's plan and in faith that, whatever the outcome, they will be all right. Some report being at odds with God for allowing their baby to be thrust out of the womb and to experience the pain of prematurity. Among those who had previously rejected the faith of their childhood, many reclaim some aspect of it as their own again; others turn to new beliefs. Most premie parents report finding solace in the prayers offered up by persons of all faiths and from across the globe, a common experience that they find comforting. For parents who cannot hold onto a God concept in the midst of their trials, many are drawn to look for the good in humankind and to the strength of modern medicine.

Having a premature baby, irrespective of gestational age or risk of complications, often leaves parents feeling completely out of control and at the mercy of their maker. This single event can cause even those with the strongest faith to examine what it is they truly believe and to scrutinize the

* WT Cummings. Field sermon, Bataan, 1942.

foundations of those beliefs. They often report that their faith is strengthened in the process. Being acutely aware that life is not in their control causes many premie parents to humbly look upward or outward in search of much needed strength for the premie journey.

In reflecting on how having a premature baby affected their spirituality, a few moms and dads shared openly with me about a topic that is often viewed as private. The following is a sampling of the thoughts and struggles these parents shared about their spirituality in response to having a premature baby:

> When [my baby] was born, all of a sudden, with no warning, after a seemingly "normal" and uneventful pregnancy, I had a flood of all those questions: *Why* did this happen? Was I being punished for something? How could a compassionate God allow this to happen?… After lots of reading and soul searching, my husband and I both came to believe that [our baby's] traumatic birth happened for a reason, and it may take us a while to figure out what that reason was, but it made more sense than "being punished for something." *—Sally*

> Sometimes I still get mad at God for doing this to my little guy and I get mad that he is continuing to struggle. But I always remind myself that God must have a lot of faith in me that I can handle it.… The premie experience has had two very different effects on my faith. One…that I can make it with God's help, and…[two] that life does not make sense…that life is not fair. *—Maureen*

> My faith was that I could get through each day with the presence of love and care from God and that my assurance from God was that I would get through this trauma.… I felt more peace and reassurance that all would be well, no matter what the outcome of her early birth, that I would be able to come through the experience intact, no matter what extreme emotions and events took place. *—Cathy*

> In a sense, I was in touch with a higher power, although not a distinctive god-type one. It was just that I absolutely had to surrender control. There was nothing

I could do to change what was happening. [My baby] would either die or he wouldn't, and I knew, finally, that I would have to accept either outcome. I think, previous to that experience, I had always believed that I could change any situation I didn't like. I had even tricked myself into believing that I had caused or allowed his premature birth. But when his intestine ruptured and we came close to losing him, I finally knew that I was really just one little person, gripping tightly for control in a world she couldn't possibly control or even really understand. It was humbling. —*Eva*

We found our spirituality to have grown tremendously. I nearly died when Caitlin was born.… The doctors basically didn't think I would make it; the hospital pastor took some pictures of her and brought them down to me. I *do* remember someone showing me pictures and saying, "This is your daughter and she needs you very much."… After that I began to stabilize. I truly believe that God sent that pastor to me to help save my life…the docs had already told my husband that it "was out of their hands." I know [God] reached out to me that day and I feel His presence all the time. —*Cindy*

How odd it was that we did not pray more.… One reason I think is that for me to keep my sanity, I had to have strong faith in the doctors and nurses that were treating my son. —*Lisa*

I had a sense that [my daughter] had a calling to accomplish on this earth. My fear was that her calling may take hours, days, or months to accomplish, rather than 60 to 70 years. —*Greg*

We had signs from the Shining Ones while there. At first light Monday morning,…there appeared a raven on the windowsill, where previously there had been only pigeons. This raven crowed three times and flew off. Shortly thereafter, Conal was born.… Ravens are sacred in our religious tradition, a symbol of strength and battle. The number three is also sacred. Mark took this as a sign from the Morrigan, a battle goddess whose symbol is the raven, that everything would be well. —*Sherilyn*

Our faith saw us through that long hospital stay and continues to carry us now that [our son] is gone, but it certainly hasn't taken away the bumps and bruises. I can say that all of this is God's will, but I believe He still feels our pain and understands when I need to scream out at that Will and wish it were otherwise. I don't think God could be God and only allow the good things to happen to us. How else could we understand joy if we didn't understand sorrow? *—Laurel*

When my baby was born early, it reminded me that I wasn't in control, but God was. Yet, I was scared by the fact that it didn't necessarily mean my baby would live or be unscathed. *—John*

While I knew that being angry would be a natural emotion, I had no anger at God. Not because I was afraid He couldn't handle my anger, God is bigger than that, but because the bible says, "God knew us even before we were formed in our mother's womb." I was anchored by that fact, which meant that God knew my baby *and* knew he would be early. My faith is in Jesus, whom I know as a loving, compassionate, intimate, and all-powerful God. He knows what is best for my baby, and He is our greatest advocate. On some days, I have to remind myself about that, but in the end, it always brings me peace. *—Danielle*

When parents are faced with the crisis of their baby's premature birth, they experience their lives suddenly spinning out of control. This often leaves them feeling helpless and powerless. The intensity of these emotions seems to compel parents to search for help and strength in new ways, and many find it in some form of spirituality.

Prior to the birth of my baby, my experience of spirituality could be described as…

Were your spiritual beliefs challenged as a result of having a premie? If so, in what way?

How have you reconciled these challenges?

Spiritually speaking, the concerns I continue to struggle with are…

Did you consider your baby's premature birth a punishment or wrath from God?

If you believe that your baby's premature birth was for some purpose, were you able to express dissatisfaction with this "means to an end"?

If you believe that your baby's premature birth was for some purpose, do you also believe that you have a role to play in bringing this purpose to fruition?

Did you ever fear that a shortened life span was God's plan for your baby's life? What were your thoughts and feelings about this?

Is there room, within the confines of your belief, to express anger, rage, sadness, fear, hopelessness, or resignation about your baby being premature?

Many persons engage in some form of bargaining with God when they face a crisis. Did you find yourself doing this? If so, what did you bargain for?

Have you been able to make sense of your baby's premature birth within the context of your spiritual beliefs? If so, how?

Did you experience any "signs" that you interpreted as meaningful with regard to your baby's prematurity? If so, describe them.

Has your belief system or faith changed as a result of having your baby prematurely?

The words or actions of others that moved me spiritually were…

I have found spiritual strength for the premie journey in…

In the midst of the crisis of having a premature baby, are there things for which you offered thanks?

Notes

Notes

Chapter Nine

Partners and Their Ways of Coping

Although partners who are anticipating the birth of their baby may feel very close to each other and may see this pregnancy as the most important unifying event in their relationship, their respective responses to its abrupt ending may be anything but unified. You may have been drawn to your partner because of your similarities, but undoubtedly there are also differences, and it is common for times of crisis to underscore these differences. Although how we each respond is not specific to gender, it does seem that partners often respond in complimentary, though sometimes conflicting, ways. One parent may feel unable to cope, completely immersed in the emotion of it all, while the other parent remains the rock of Gibraltar, attending to every detail and seemingly unscathed by the crisis of their baby's precarious arrival. One parent may feel the need to be strong for and take care of the other, while the other wishes for more open communication between them. One parent may be an "information hound," devouring all the medical terminology and outcome predictions, while the other may respond in total optimism, seeing their baby as relatively healthy without feeling the need to dwell on what "might be."

It is not uncommon during the premie journey for partners to find that their ways of coping cause some distress to their mate. Having a premature baby is a crisis, but it can be a different crisis to each parent. Each perceives the crisis through a uniquely filtered lens, focusing on what he or she perceives to be the critical issues. Likewise, both respond to the crisis as they come to understand it, in their own unique manners. In this regard, it is not uncommon for parents to experience some resentment that their partner is not responding to the situation just like they are or is not responding in ways they feel they need. Those who have a desire to process their emotions may feel that their partner is detached or in denial. Those who have a need to consider all the options and likely outcomes may feel their partner is defensive or naïve. The demands, both physical and emotional, made on premie parents during their baby's early stages and subsequent growth periods can place a strain on even the strongest bonds.

In this environment, parents are stretched to find the time and energy necessary to work through their differences, hurt, anger, disappointment, and resentment. Yet when parents are able to carve out the time and muster the energy necessary to address issues, to be heard, to make changes, and, when necessary, to agree to disagree, they find that the family bond is strengthened.

Contemplate how you and your partner have coped with the premie journey.

Describe the way you responded emotionally to your baby's early birth.

What actions did you take to cope with your baby's early birth and hospitalization?

Describe the way your partner responded emotionally to your baby's early birth.

What actions did your partner take to cope with your baby's early birth and hospitalization?

Did you and your partner struggle with similar issues in regard to your baby's prematurity, or were they different?

Were your coping styles complimentary? If so, how?

Were your coping styles in conflict? If so, how?

What I needed from my partner at this time was…

What I wish I could have given to my partner was…

What I wish my partner could have understood was…

The crisis of having our baby prematurely caused our relationship to…

As a result of this crisis, what I have learned about my partner is that he or she…

As a result of this crisis, what my partner has likely learned about me is that I…

I appreciate most the way my partner…

Do you wish you could be more like your partner in some ways? If so, how? Have you shared this with your partner?

Have your respective coping strategies continued as before, or have they changed over time?

As a result of your baby's premature birth, are there areas of difficulty in your relationship that have not been resolved?

Are there things you really wanted your partner to know, but that have gone unsaid?

What I still need to talk to my partner about is...

Notes

Chapter Ten

When Baby Is Not First-Born: Heart and Home Divided

Couples report that beginning the premie journey when they are already parents equips them with vital tools. One mom shared, "I was glad to learn I was having a boy because I knew how to parent a boy, but I didn't know how to parent a premie. Yet, being a mom already gave me a sense of confidence in my ability to learn how to nurture my premie and give him, or get for him, all that he would need." Most seasoned parents experience fewer, albeit different, concerns about their ability to nurture, about knowing what it is to be a parent, about juggling care for self with care for others, and to some extent about knowing how to read their baby's cues than first-time parents do. They likely have had some experience with the ups and downs, the frights and joys, that come with being a caregiver. Parents have reported that even the nursing staff in the NICU seemed to treat them differently because they were "veterans."

However, having children at home when a premie is born also adds complications. First-time parents may be more free to spend their time giving their premie undivided attention, but parents with children at home are pulled in different directions. They often feel that they are neglecting their other children because visiting a premie in the NICU most often means being separated from them. One mom shared, "When I was in the NICU, my heart was breaking to be at home with my other children, and when I was at home, my heart was breaking to be with my premie. It was difficult to ever feel whole." Caring for a premie in the NICU causes drastic changes in the usual routine. By necessity, family schedules have to be altered if parents are to spend time bonding and caring for their premie. Already struggling to balance work, marriage, and family life, parents now also have to juggle hospital visitations and keeping close friends and family abreast of their baby's condition.

Although parents might have otherwise been able to incorporate their new baby into their usual family routine, not having the baby at home brings unique challenges. Balancing the demands of home while being away, arranging new forms of child care, traveling to and from the hospital, making alternate living arrangements, and attending to the physical, social, and emotional needs of their older children are but a few of the challenges that must be met. All these demands occur while also having to deal with one's own emotional reaction to the trauma of having a premie. Although the logistics of change are difficult, the greatest burden seems to be on the heart. It is impossible to be in two places at the same time and impossible to give to one's children equally. Premie parents must contend with caring for their children in separate homes and with divided hearts.

Record your experience, both practical and emotional, of your own "heart and home divided."

How have you managed parenting on two different fronts?

Who was available to help you with this process?

How often were you able to visit with your premie in the NICU?

What arrangements were needed in order to accommodate your visiting schedule?

Do you live near the hospital? Or did you have to commute? How was this helpful or cumbersome?

Did you need to make alternative living arrangements? Was anyone helpful in this process?

What sibling schedules did you have to manage or juggle?

Did you need to make alternative child care arrangements? How was this managed?

Emotionally, I found all of this to be…

Did your children experience any developmental regression during this time, such as moodiness, bed wetting, or separation anxiety?

Did your children demonstrate any stress reactions, such as nightmares or nail biting?

What discussions have you had with your children about their premie sibling and about the disruption of life as they knew it?

What were their thoughts, concerns, and fears about you being away during visits with your baby?

What were their thoughts, concerns, and fears about their baby brother or sister?

What assurances were you able to give your children?

Were your other children able to visit with the baby? If so, what was their emotional reaction?

Was there a need to respond to their reaction? If so, what helped them?

How did you attend to your children's needs while you were at the hospital? For example, did you leave notes for them, call frequently, or prepare special meals ahead of time?

In order to feel connected with my baby when I was at home, I…

How did you cope with not being able to attend to all your children's needs equally?

What family traditions did you maintain during your baby's stay in the NICU?

Did you find ways to include your baby in family traditions?

Were there things you did that helped older siblings cope with all the changes? If so, what?

The most difficult of all the adjustments I had to make was…

Are there things you wish you had done differently? If so, describe them.

Are there things that you did with which you are pleased? If so, describe them.

Notes

Chapter Eleven

Homeward Bound: Ready or Not, Here I Come!

Premies come into the world before their time, and no matter how much forewarning parents have, it is always too soon. These babies spend seemingly endless days in the NICU, often gestating there the length of time they would have spent *in utero.* Parents wait for their baby to heal and then to grow. Many wonder if the day will ever come when they will be able to take their baby home. One day, the wait *is* over. Then the time to take their baby home can seem too soon! Although parents have long been anxious to leave the NICU, they may secretly wonder if they are ready to care for their baby all on their own.

When the word *discharge* is spoken, parents often have mixed emotions. To be sure, they are elated that their baby is well enough to go home and relieved beyond compare to be leaving the NICU, but many are also fearful that they are now fully in charge of their premie. Some parents report feeling anxious about going home without any monitors on which to rely. They are afraid that if their baby has "As and Bs," they won't know about it. Others are thankful to be transporting monitors home with the baby. One mom said, "If I couldn't take the nurses home with me, at least I had the monitor that would beep if anything went wrong." Still others want no reminder that their baby was so ill. Consequently, when the baby is sent home on oxygen or monitors, they report experiencing feelings of failure, however unrealistic, because their baby needs more than they could provide by themselves.

The transition from hospital to home is accompanied by the transition from parent helper to solo parent. The time has come when the parents' decision is the final decision. Sleep schedules, feedings, massage, or kangaroo care are now determined as parents deem it best for the baby. Although parents have waited eagerly for this time to come, there has been no easing into the job, no extensive "on-the-job training." The change from assisting with care to being the full-time caregiver, no matter how keenly longed for, can be anxiety producing. However, despite the apprehension, parents quickly learn that their time spent in the NICU has helped prepare them for their job at home.

The NICU is a training ground for parents. Caring for their baby in the hospital helps parents learn to read their baby's cues, to recognize what their baby needs, to understand their baby's likes and dislikes—in short, it helps them come to know their baby's personality. It is important for parents to recognize that once they get their baby home, they do not have to continue on this journey alone. Although the baton has been passed, most NICU nurses welcome, if not encourage, calls from moms and dads to help ease the transition to home care. Pediatricians, lactation consultants, hospital pediatric dieticians, and local developmental specialists are also available to parents in need of information or simple reassurance. Although they may wonder if they're ready to take on their premie's full care, parents can rest assured that they *do* have what it takes to provide for their baby or to obtain all that he or she will need.

Parents should also remember that although the NICU is comforting because state-of-the-art technology and medical expertise is at hand, it is not the place for complete healing. Generally speaking, it is not until babies are home that they begin to thrive. When moved to the nurturing environment of home, babies are surrounded with the sights, sounds, and smells of those who love them. Home is the place where your baby can be fed, held, sung to, talked with, and otherwise nurtured around the clock. When your baby is basked in the sunlight and orchestra of your loving family, healing and thriving will follow.

Reflect on your homeward bound experience.

When I heard that my baby was ready to come home, I responded by…

I prepared emotionally for my baby's homecoming by…

How did you prepare physically for your baby's homecoming? For instance, did you decorate a nursery, room in with your baby, or obtain special training?

Describe your baby's homecoming.

Describe your first day and night at home with your baby.

How old was your baby when discharged from the NICU? How much did your baby weigh?

Did your baby come home on monitors or oxygen? What was your reaction to the need for this equipment in your home?

Describe your baby's initial sleep and feeding schedule.

Where did your baby sleep at first?

What was your and your partner's sleep schedule like when your baby first came home?

Did your baby have difficulty adjusting to the change from hospital to home environment?

How did you help your baby adjust to life at home?

Was anyone available to help you? If so, who, and in what ways did they help?

Were your baby's first few days at home different than you expected? If so, how?

Did you or your partner do kangaroo care at home? If so, describe your experience.

Did you or your partner do infant massage with your baby? If so, describe your experience.

Did you change or attempt to change your baby's schedule in any way? If so, how and why?

Were you able to feed your baby in the manner you had hoped, such as complete breastfeeding, expressed breast milk with supplements, or bottle feeding?

What were your main concerns when your baby first arrived at home? Have these concerns changed any since then?

How concerned were you about needing to keep your baby free of germs? Did this alter your lifestyle in any way?

How did you deal with visitors initially? Has this changed with the passage of time?

Did you celebrate your baby's homecoming? If so, when and how?

Did your baby have any feeding difficulties?

Did you have concerns about your baby's health? If so, have those concerns changed since your baby first came home?

What was your reaction to leaving the medical staff who cared for you and your baby?

Did you carry over any of the hospital routines, such as charting your baby's weight, medications, or progress?

Have you left your baby with child care to resume work or to spend time alone with your partner? What has this been like for you?

Now that you are all home, how have you begun to heal and thrive?

Notes

Notes

Chapter Twelve
Coping with Complications

Parents of premature babies are well aware how vulnerable their children are to potential health problems as they grow and develop. Some premies are discharged from the NICU with a diagnosis that guarantees certain short- or long-term complications. Although hospital staff do their best to prepare parents for the potential difficulties ahead, only time reveals the full extent of medical challenges they may face with their child. Such a host of unknowns only intensifies parents' anxiety. One mom expressed concern about her child's development: "It's so hard not knowing what the future holds for my daughter. I wonder if she'll ever walk on her own and how she'll interact with others. I wish we had some answers, but we just have to wait."

A diagnosis can bring a sense of relief to parents by resolving some of the uncertainties about their child's condition. It allows parents to redirect their energy toward obtaining productive remedies. But a diagnosis can also be devastating, no matter when it's received or how much warning one has. When a diagnosis or prognosis is confirmed, parents often relive the grief they first experienced with their baby's premature birth, and they may struggle with lingering feelings of guilt as their child's health complications become more evident. Denial of the diagnosis is common, but it often progresses to the question "Why me?" Parents mourn the loss of the child they thought they would have and grieve the loss of experiences their child will never participate in or excel at. They wrestle with questions such as "If I had done this differently, would this have happened?" The mother of a four-year-old premie who now needs glasses says, "I feel horribly guilty that she has to wear them. If she hadn't been premature, would she need them? Maybe, maybe not, but I know now it is a result of the ROP, so I feel guilty! Sometimes those small premie issues can sneak up on you and really throw you a curve."

The types and degrees of complications stemming from a premature birth range anywhere from feeding issues, motor coordination, and mental, visual, and verbal impairments to serious respiratory and heart problems. Use of monitors, oxygen tanks, nebulizers, tracheostomy equipment, home nurses, and physical, occupational, or speech therapists can become routine as parents concentrate on caring for their child with special needs. Life may seem like one prolonged doctor's appointment. Premie parents often compare life to a "roller coaster" and talk about "taking one day at a time." One mom shared, "No day is normal and it probably never will be." Another stated, "I celebrate what he can do, and [I] don't cry over what he can't do." Yet, she also disclosed that she does cry at times when faced with the reality of seeing her child's differences. When parents observe children the same age as their child mastering skills their premie is far from attaining, they may make false comparisons that bring up feelings of guilt and sadness. However, when this happens, parents need to pause and remind themselves that their child is, as one mom put it, "her own person." And although they are eager for their child to reach each milestone, anxiously wondering if he or she will make it, parents must come to appreciate what their child has achieved and delight in the progress made. If parents are wise, they will learn to allow their child to develop at his or her own pace, defining what is "normal" on an individual basis.

Other issues become important as a child's health issues become more clear. First, when dealing with their child's medical and developmental issues, parents often learn to become strong advocates for their child. Though a multitude of professionals may be involved in making decisions regarding the well-being of children with special needs, parents know their own child best. When properly informed, they are the best guardians of their child's interests when dealing with insurance companies, doctors, therapists, and schools. At first, the job of advocate can seem all-consuming for parents. As they learn this vital role, which requires time and persistence in communicating their child's needs, services made available to their child will become better tailored to their special circumstances.

Additionally, parents with other children often wonder how these siblings will be affected by the disproportionate amount of physical and emotional energy directed toward the child with disabilities. Although some children at times feel neglected by their parents and embarrassed about their sibling's condition, these responses are by no means the rule. On the contrary, one mother shared that the situation "made the other siblings more sensitive and compassionate and blind to such differences." Turning difficulties into a positive life experience, she noted that "the other children participated in our daughter's care, stimulating her development and sharing pride in her progress."

Caring for a child with disabilities can be physically, emotionally, and financially challenging, as parents adjust to the pain of unfulfilled expectations and loss. However, through effective advocacy and sibling involvement, they are likely to discover surprising joys and rewards in the very challenges of raising a child with special needs.

Tell how your've coped with your child's complications.

Describe the extent of your child's complications.

When were you first aware that your child would have complications?

How were you told this news, and how prepared were you to hear it?

What was your reaction to hearing of your child's complications?

What was your partner's reaction?

Did you have concerns about your child before the professionals took notice? If so, how did you go about getting these concerns addressed? How did you feel about this process?

I have coped with the uncertainties of the future by…

My greatest fears with regard to my child's medical condition are…

Have you had any guilt about your child's disabilities? If so, describe your feelings.

How have others reacted to your child's disabilities?

What has been your response to these reactions or comments?

How have you grieved the pain of unfulfilled expectations and loss?

What is your strategy for coping with the re-emergence of old emotions that you thought you had resolved?

Has anyone among your family or friends been in denial regarding your child's condition or diagnosis? If so, how was this denial expressed?

Who or what has offered you the greatest support?

What adjustments have you had to make in your life because of your child's special needs?

How has your relationship with your partner been affected? What adjustments have been made?

How have your other children been affected?

What adjustments have they had to make?

Have you received any conflicting information about your child's treatment plans or prognosis?

Have you ever felt afraid to ask or repeat a question of a health care professional to ensure that you understood the information? If so, how have you—or how might you—quell this fear?

What has been your experience in dealing with doctors, therapists, and school personnel in regard to your child's special needs?

Were you ever labeled or made to feel like you are "an overprotective parent"?

In what ways have you needed to be an advocate for your child? What has this experience been like for you?

Describe some highlights in your child's progress.

Describe some disappointments in your child's progress.

What kind of financial adjustments have you needed to make because of your child's disability?

What struggles have you faced in finding child care or respite care? Who or what has supported you in this effort?

How have the challenges of caring for your child changed as your child has grown?

What have you learned about yourself as a result of meeting the demands of your child's condition?

What has your child taught you through this experience?

Notes

Notes

Notes

Chapter Thirteen

Another Baby? To Have or Not to Have

After having a premie, parents will never look upon pregnancy in the same way again. The harsh reality that a pregnancy has ended before its optimum time ushers in a permanent change in thinking about pregnancy. One mom wrote, "The thing about having a premie is that the excitement and expectation in your future pregnancies is ruined." For some parents, thinking about whether or not to have another baby occurs rather quickly. One mom shared, "While I was on the OR table in the middle of my premie's C-section, I said to myself emphatically, 'I *never* want to go through this again.'" For others, having another baby may be something they don't even consider until the initial storm of their premie's birth is over. For still others, it may not occur until their premie is no longer a baby. One dad shared, "It wasn't until our baby was walking and thriving that we felt ready to have another one."

Perhaps the most obvious way one's ideal of pregnancy changes after a premature birth is in the automatic question that seems to follow the thought of a subsequent pregnancy: Will another baby be at risk for prematurity? Mothers report fear that their bodies—their uterus, their cervix, or their immune system—will fail them again, and as a result, they will fail a new baby. One mom shared, "I just couldn't cope with the thought of ever being pregnant again and knowing that I was at risk for another premature delivery. My premie would need all I could give him." Others are more optimistically certain that, with their current knowledge, they would be equipped to watch for early signs of trouble. They are hopeful that using early intervention strategies would yield a better outcome for subsequent pregnancies.

For some parents, the thought of another pregnancy brings with it a sense of resolve. Many moms disclose that their desire to have another baby is intertwined with their need to have a pregnancy go to term and to have a birth that more closely resembles what their ideal had been. In this respect, a new pregnancy offers the hope of some repair—a chance to complete that which previously came to a screeching halt. One mom, whose premature boys were now in early and middle adolescence, noted, "I still want to be pregnant again so that I can complete a pregnancy....[When both of my boys were born] I still had planning to do, and my bags weren't even packed." Even for premie parents whose subsequent deliveries are premature, these later pregnancies can represent repair, although in a different manner. Being somewhat familiar with how this scenario might play out and having in mind what they want to be different can equip and empower parents to more satisfactorily navigate their next premie journey.

Share what thoughts you've entertained regarding future pregnancies.

Do you fear having another premature delivery?

Is this fear dampening your desire for another baby?

Have you entertained thoughts that your body—your uterus, your cervix, your immune system—might "fail" you again?

Are you aware of any underlying reasons in your desire to have another baby, such as to make up for what you missed out on with your premie or to have a more ideal pregnancy and birth?

Do you entertain thoughts that it would be selfish of you to have another baby, if that baby were to be premature?

If a subsequent baby were to be born prematurely, would you blame yourself for bringing that baby into the world and for causing him or her pain?

If a subsequent baby has been born prematurely, did you blame yourself for bringing that baby into the world and for causing him or her pain?

What sense have you made of your premie's early birth? How have you allowed yourself to grieve the loss of your ideal pregnancy and birthing experience?

What do you need to do emotionally to clear the passage for subsequent pregnancies?

Did you, or do you, need to forgive yourself or your body for a less-than-perfect pregnancy and delivery?

What knowledge do you have now that will help you recognize any early indicators of trouble?

My hope for a subsequent pregnancy is that it would be…

If you have had a postpremie pregnancy:

When I found out I was pregnant again, my reaction was…

My partner's reaction was…

In what ways did having a premie affect the later pregnancy?

I took some precautionary measures during this pregnancy, including…

This pregnancy and delivery were different from the pregnancy and delivery of my premie in that…

Did this later pregnancy and delivery bring about healing? If so, describe how this healing occurred.

Notes

Notes

Notes

Chapter Fourteen

Looking Back Over the Years: Will I Ever Be Done with This?

When parents are in the beginning stages of the premie journey, they can find it difficult to imagine anything beyond their current struggle. Yet there *is* a future in store for them and their families. For parents grieving the death of their premie, the future will include their baby, who will forever be a part of them, a part of their family history. For those who will watch their premie grow, the premie journey does not end upon discharge from the NICU. Instead, it continues to evolve. For some, it requires minimum amounts of extra energy; for others, it becomes the focal point of their lives thereafter. Many parents at various stages of this journey will ask the question: "When will I be over this?" However, over time, they come to rephrase the question, later asking: "Will I ever be done with this?" The subtle change in wording of that poignant question reflects the ongoing process that is the premie journey.

Questioning when their grief will stop may be prompted by parents' perception that others have lost interest in supporting their grief and are now wanting, even expecting, them to "get on with their lives." Moms and dads themselves want to be able to "get over this" and resume life as it used to be, or as they dreamed it would be. Yet, at any time, the emotions they once felt in the NICU can be triggered, and parents find themselves reliving the traumatic feelings once associated with their child's early birth. This kind of experience often leads parents to question the extent of their own healing.

Experts in the field of trauma describe the healing of grief as a process. It is not a one-time event that is successfully cured. Rather, it is a process through which one moves, a journey of active grieving and support, as over time, memories are accompanied by less intense emotions. Parents may feel some sadness that things were, or are, less than ideal for their precious premie. Yet, they do come to find peace and resolve in the understanding that this is their journey. Many report that this process is not linear and that these periods of resolve are interrupted by times of renewed grief. They do note, however, that the peaceful periods grow steadily longer.

The anniversary of the onset of labor, the baby's birth, the due date, or discharge from the NICU, or even simply driving by the hospital, can trigger the flood of emotions that once characterized the NICU experience. These times often lead to a reworking of grief, guilt, anger, sadness, and loss. It is likely, however, that gradually these emotions will be experienced in a different manner. Time has begun to heal these wounds. And as parents' reactions to the triggering events become less intense, they may find that these events now serve as reminders that prompt feelings of gratitude. Parents are thankful for the life of their premie, thankful for his or her presence in their lives. They have begun to make peace with the premie journey, recognizing that their lives are forever changed because of this birth. This is the process of healing.

The following section is provided to give you a place to write a birthday letter to your premie. This can become a meaningful tradition that also gives you a forum for evaluating the journey that you and your child have navigated thus far. You may choose to write a summary of your premie's past year, the challenges and triumphs, your own joys and trials as you've watched your child grow, your hopes and dreams for your premie, or anything else you'd like him or her to know. If your infant is deceased, you may want to write a letter in his or her memory.

First-Year Memories:

175

Second-Year Memories:

Third-Year Memories:

Fourth-Year Memories:

Fifth-Year Memories:

Notes

Appendix A
Parents' Log

Record daily notes, pertinent information, or questions to be adressed with others.

Date: ______________ Subject: ______________

Note:

Date: ______________ Subject: ______________

Note:

Date: ______________ Subject: ______________

Note:

Date: ______________ Subject: ______________

Note:

Date: ______________ Subject: ______________

Note:

Date: ______________ Subject: ______________

Note:

Date: ______________ Subject: ______________

Note:

Date: ______________________ Subject: ______________________________

Note:

____

____

____

Date: ______________________ Subject: ______________________________

Note:

____

____

____

Date: ______________________ Subject: ______________________________

Note:

____

____

____

Date: ______________________ Subject: ______________________________

Note:

____

____

____

Date: ______________ Subject: ______________

Note:

____

____

____

Date: ______________ Subject: ______________

Note:

____

____

____

Date: ______________ Subject: ______________

Note:

____

____

____

Date: ______________ Subject: ______________

Note:

____

____

____

Date: ______________ Subject: ______________

Note:

Date: ______________ Subject: ______________

Note:

Date: ______________ Subject: ______________

Note:

Date: ______________ Subject: ______________

Note:

Date: Subject:

Note:

Date: Subject:

Note:

Date: Subject:

Note:

Date: Subject:

Note:

Appendix B

Baby's Diary

Date	Baby's Weight	Note

Date	Baby's Weight	Note

Date	Baby's Weight	Note

Date	Baby's Weight	Note

Date	Baby's Weight	Note

Date	Baby's Weight	Note

Appendix C
Photo and Mementos Pocket

Appendix C
Photo and Mementos Pocket

Appendix D
Parent Resources

Helpful Reading

Abbott Northwestern Hospital. 1993. *A Fragile Beginning: Parenting Your Early Baby*. Minneapolis, Minnesota: Abbott Northwestern Hospital, 612-863-5964.

Barsuhn R. 1996. *Growing Sophia: The Story of a Premature Birth.* St. Paul, Minnesota: A Place To Remember.

Davis DL. 1999. *Empty Cradle, Broken Heart: Surviving the Death of Your Baby.* Golden, Colorado: Fulcrum.

Davis DL, and Stein MT. In press. *The Emotional Journey of Parenting Your Premature Baby: A Book of Hope and Healing.* Santa Rosa, California: NICU Ink.

Hussey-Gardner B. 1996. *Understanding My Signals: Help for Parents of Premature Infants.* Palo Alto, California: VORT. (This publication may be obtained through a health care provider.)

Ludington-Hoe S. 2001. *Kangaroo Care: The Best You Can Do for Your Premature Infant.* New York: Bantam Books.

Tracy AE, and Maroney DI. 1999. *Your Premature Baby and Child: Helpful Answers and Advice for Parents.* New York: Berkley Publishing Group.

Walker M. 1994. 1998. *Breastfeeding Your Premature or Special Care Baby: A Practice Guide for Nursing the Tiny Baby,* 4th ed. Lactation Associates, 254 Conant Road, Weston, MA 02194.

Zaichkin J. 1996. *Newborn Intensive Care: What Every Parent Needs to Know.* Santa Rosa, California: NICU Ink.

On-line Support and Information

Resources for Parents of Premies: http://members.aol.com/maraim/premie.htm
Coalition for Prematurity Awareness: www.premieawareness.org
Parents of Premature Babies, Inc. (Preemie-L): www.preemie-L.org
Newborns in Need, Inc.: www.newbornsinneed.org
The Premie Store and More: www.premie.com
Premie dolls: www.macatawa.org/~eding/dolls.html

Helping Older Siblings Cope

The authors wish to thank Kelsey and Amanda Rathbun and Zachary Hacker for their invaluable assistance in compiling the information included in this section.

- Talk with your children about what has happened and answer their questions.
- Listen to your children's concerns and respond to them honestly, considering their developmental level in your response.
- Don't promise your children anything you cannot deliver, such as "The baby will be fine."
- Understand that it will be hard for your children when mom or dad go to visit the baby in the hospital.
- Ask your children to tell you what kinds of things might make this easier, and do those things that you are able.
- Expect developmental regressions such as increased crying, clinging, separation anxiety, moodiness, quick temper, bed-wetting, or nightmares; and be patient and nurturing with your children.
- Ask your children to draw pictures "about the baby" and then to tell you about their drawings. These drawings may reveal a lot about their thoughts and fears concerning you and the baby.
- Let your children know they are special and that you are thinking of them by:
  - Having them visit with the baby in the NICU as often as they desire and are able
  - Providing activities and caregivers they enjoy while they wait during your NICU visits

- Spending special time with them following a visit to the NICU (e.g., eating in the hospital cafeteria or feeding ducks in a pond)
- Letting them help with any part of the "cares" that they are old enough to handle, even if only handing you a blanket
- Having them choose a special item of clothing for the baby
- Having them select a photo of themselves to be placed in the baby's isolette
- Purchasing or giving them something special as a gift from the baby
- Writing them a note from the baby
- Calling them and sending them mail if you must be away from them
- Trying to arrange child care in their own home and always with the same caregiver, if possible, if you must be away from them
- Maintaining as much of their routine as possible
- Having a regular day or weekend at home with them and letting them be the focus of your attention
- Doing anything else you know that would be meaningful to them